Essential Oils: Recipes For DIY Aromatherapy

Complete Guide for Weight Loss, Beauty, and Health for Beginners and Experts Alike

By Emilia Hayes

Table of Contents

Chapter 10: Pests -The Uninvited Guests

Conclusion

Carrier Oils Used in this Book

Disclaimer

The oils and blends listed are not intended to replace a physician's care when needed. We do not claim that the oils will heal or cure any ailments, only that they may aid in the process.

CAUTION: Do not use oils on children, the elderly, pregnant, or lactating women without the approval of a physician. Also, research oils and read prescription inserts to learn if any of the prescriptions or over the counter drugs that you take will be counteracted or cause side effects when the oils are used. Finally, do not ingest any essential oil, or carrier oil, unless the label clearly states that the oil can be taken internally. Serious side effects may occur.

Essential Oils

Recipes for DIY Aromatherapy

Introduction

I stood in the garage doorway begging my rollerblading son to turn down the volume on his boom box. The music blared so loudly, I could scarcely hear my own voice. Wham! My thumb was smashed in the doorjamb. Blood oozed from the top and sides of my thumbnail. I wailed in pain and stuck my thumb into my mouth. What just happened? I turned to see my youngest son, standing behind me, staring. Unaware that I had been standing in the doorway, he attempted to slam out the deafening music so he could concentrate on his homework. We both cried. He cried because he hadn't intended to hurt me, and I cried because it hurt so badly! In all reality, it was my fault. I mean, who stands in any doorway with their thumb in the doorjamb? Not me! At least, not anymore!

Months later, my nail grew out, yet a deep crevice remained in my thumb. I followed my doctor's treatment, with no improvement. There was nothing left to do except put up with that ugly thumb of many colors. Through the years my thumbnail continued to change colors and fungus developed in the hole in my thumb. It totally grossed me out.

Ten years later, a friend who had recently become a distributer of essential oils suggested I try a concoction of oils to heal my thumb. I hesitantly agreed. What did I have to lose? After a few months, my thumb healed, the fungus disappeared, and even the gaping hole in my nail filled in. You guessed it; I am now a believer in essential oils. I am not promising that you would have the same result, but it worked for me, and, if the fungus, discoloration and hole return, I now have the know-how to treat my thumb.

This leads us to three obvious questions:

1.   What is an essential oil?

2.   Are essential oils a fad?

3.   What can essential oils do for me?

What is an Essential Oil?

As the crisp, spring breeze blew through Peter's lovely English flower garden in Long Stratton, England, the brilliant fragrances of roses, geranium, jasmine and lavender filled the sweet morning air. His exquisite herb garden was just as beautiful, with scents of marjoram, mint, oregano, rosemary, thyme and basil. "To the Englishman, his gardens are his pride," he told us, as he shooed a white rabbit from the herb garden. "The house is merely a living space."

I relive that wisp of fragrant breeze from Peter's glorious gardens each day as I raise the lid of my wooden box that holds my essential oils.

Essential oils are the gifts of the earth Mother Nature has blessed us with. Their very aroma creates a sensory experience. An essential oil is the "essence" of volatile liquids extracted through distillation or cold pressing of the seeds, roots, bark, stems, leaves, flowers, fruits, or any other usable part of plants.

Without getting too scientific, as many publications and search engines will lead you to those answers, I will simply clarify that essential oils stimulate physical, emotional and spiritual healing.

With the types and varieties of essential oils available, the benefits include, but are not limited to: powerful antioxidants which counterbalance free radicals; liver support in detoxifying the blood; destroying many harmful bacteria and viruses; and providing immune system support. They may promote antibacterial, antifungal, anti-infectious, antimicrobial, antitumor, anti-parasitic, antiviral and antiseptic properties, depending on which oil you are using.

Are Essential Oils a Fad?

Cave paintings found in Lascaux, France, suggest that medicinal plants were used in 18,000. B. C. E. Egyptian papyri and Chinese manuscripts report use of aromatics for healing purposes thousands of years ago. The Bible and Torah refer to ointments, incense and aromatics. Additional records show that ancient civilizations using aromatic oils include Greece, Rome, Israel, Arabia, Persia and Europe. Other ancient uses of essential oils, or aromatic oils, include food preparation, perfumery and beauty treatments. For thousands of years oils have been used to spiritually and emotionally uplift the psyche, and to ward off evil spirits. In many cultures, specific precious oils were reserved for deity and pharaohs. In the showing of respect, King

Tutankhamen's tomb was graced with alabaster jars of aromatic oils.

Revived interest has occurred in recent decades bringing essential oils out of obscurity and into popularity. Today researchers, scientists, physicians, chemists and interested individuals are discovering positive aspects of essential oils. Many "preppers" stock up on essential oils in case medicine and doctor's care becomes scarce. Essential oils are often packed in emergency kits or backpacks, since they take up little space, yet their uses are so versatile.

What can Essential Oils do for me?

As you read through the pages of this book, you will discover the various ways essential oils can be of value. Many have been brushed lightly upon in the above paragraphs.

One of the most important things to remember as you purchase essential oils is that not all oils are created equally. Take care to research therapeutic- grade oils. The difference in the pure oils and the less quality oils lies in the distilling process or cold expression used, and whether or not a carrier oil has been added to the essential oil to dilute it. This is a practice known in the world by companies or individuals who try to pass off substandard oil when you think you are buying pure oil. The ingredient label on higher grade oils will list all ingredients, including the botanical names. These higher grade oils cost more than their second-rate replicas. Choose oils that are stored in dark-colored bottles.

A carrier oil is often used by an individual to help carry an essential oil into the skin, and to spread it over a larger area. In definition, a carrier is derived from a vegetable, wax, fat or other source that an essential oil is mixed with. Popular carriers include: fractionated coconut oil, jojoba, extra virgin olive oil, almond oil, grapeseed oil, sesame oil, soybean oil and sunflower oil. Additional carriers are also available on the market.

There are three approved ways to use essential oils.

1.   Topically – In this method the essential oil is applied directly to the skin. In most cases, a carrier oil may be used for easier spreading of the oil. As a caution, do not mix essential oils

with water, butter, vegetable oil, shortening or mineral oil when applying topically.

2.	Aromatically – Inhaling a mist of oil, or oils, is produced by diffusing in an essential oil friendly diffuser; smelling the oil directly from the bottle; or rubbing a few drops between your palms, and sniffing them occasionally as you go about your day. Do not heat oils. This may decrease their potency.

3.	Internally – Not all oils can be taken internally. Please heed this caution to study the bottle label before ingesting. A drop or two can replace some of the spices in your recipes, or add an additional flavor. A few drops in a glass pitcher of orange, lemon or peppermint, to name a few, will add a fresh taste to your water and add health benefits. Only use a glass pitcher and a glass drinking glass. Dropping a few oils into a gelatin capsule is another option for taking oil internally.

Now that we have briefly discussed essential oils, it's time to learn more about a handful of individual oils and what they can do for you. A list of essential oils used in each chapter precedes the recipes. Carriers referenced in this book are listed and described at the end of the book. Sit back, relax; a fresh, vibrant world awaits you!

Chapter 1: Lose Weight - Feel Great

After returning from our holiday in England, my husband and I both discovered we had lost a few pounds, with no desire in finding them. In touring, we walked several miles each day and skipped lunches. At that point we pledged to keep the weight off and to lose even more. Together, we started an intense diet and exercise program. I am happy to boast that I lost 33 pounds in less than a year. Since that time, I have dabbled in essential oils, and have wondered how they might have assisted me in losing the weight. Hopefully, I will never know. I am, however, maintaining the weight loss with essential oils.

The weight loss benefits of the essential oils basil, cinnamon, eucalyptus, fennel, ginger, grapefruit, lemon, peppermint, rosemary and sandalwood will be discussed in this chapter.

Basil: Used often in cooking, this spicy, herbaceous oil aids in digestion.

Cinnamon: The warm, sweet, spirited fragrance and flavor of this oil may regulate blood sugar levels and reduce inflammation.

Eucalyptus: This oil is used to increase energy and to soothe sore muscles. Its fragrance is earthy, cooling and freshening.

Fennel: This earthy, sweet fragrant oil, similar to anise, may suppress appetite, reduce weight gain, improve digestion and encourage a restful night's sleep.

Ginger: Known to improve digestion and increase energy, this oil carries a spicy, woody aroma.

Grapefruit: This citrus oil, sweet, crisp and tangy, is used to boost metabolism, curb cravings, increase energy and to reduce abdominal fat. Sun sensitivity may occur while using citrus oils. Read warning labels on bottles.

Lemon: Used often in flavoring, this clean, uplifting, citrusy oil enhances the mood, increases energy, relieves pain and suppresses weight gain. Sun sensitivity may occur while using citrus oils. Read warning labels on the bottles.

Orange: Flavors water and food with its familiar tangy taste and scent. Orange oil aids in digestion, decreases appetite and is uplifting to your mood. Sun sensitivity may occur while using citrus oils. Read warning labels on the bottle.

Peppermint: Minty, fresh and cooling, this oil is used to aid digestion, reduce appetite, increase energy and to elevate mood.

Rosemary: This oil is used to shed fat and to aid in digestion. It carries a sweet, fresh and penetrating smell.

Sandalwood: With its woody, sweet fragrance, this oil helps overcome stress eating and creates emotional balance.

Blend 1: My Workout Perk

2 drops Basil

3 drops Eucalyptus

3 drops Peppermint

2 drops Rosemary

Fractionated Coconut oil

To perk up your workout, add the four essential oils into a 10 ml roller bottle and fill remainder of the bottle with coconut oil leaving enough headspace to add the roller ball. To use, roll across your joints and the muscle groups you plan to focus on during your routine. Massage in with your hands. After your workout this mixture may relieve sore muscles.

Blend 2: Citrus Delight

5 drops of Grapefruit

3 drops of Lemon

1 drop of Orange

Stir oils into a 2 quart glass pitcher of water. Store in the fridge and drink throughout the day to suppress appetite.

Blend 3: Citrusy, Cinnamon Drink

1 drop Cinnamon

1 drop Ginger

1 drop Grapefruit

Add oils to a glass of cold water. Stir. This recipe is intended to curb appetite.

Blend 4: Spice of Life

1 drop Cinnamon

1 drop Grapefruit

2 drops Ginger

1 teaspoon Fractionated Coconut or other carrier oil

Pour carrier oil into your palm. Stir with your finger and then massage into abdomen in a circular motion, smoothing across the navel. This recipe could also be used to diffuse oils if you leave out the carrier oil and add the drops to a water-filled diffuser.

Summary

Though there is no miracle cure for weight loss, the essential oils and recipes listed are intended to aid in healthy eating and exercise. Personally, I find that adding drops of essential oils to my drinking water not only helps with curbing my appetite, but encourages me to drink more water. As far as exercise goes, if I rub essential oils on my joints and stiff muscles, I am able to work out longer and harder than when I neglect to use the oils.

Chapter 2: Skin Deep

Rosalie set up a corner shop in a rural town where she sells essential oil products. She has experimented to find the right combinations of essential oils to make sunscreens, soaps, lip balm and skin care products. Traveling around to fairs and local celebrations, she sells many homemade concoctions with repeat customers. Though Rosalie hasn't unveiled her recipes, following are some formulas that make fine skin care solutions.

Frankincense: Rich, warm and balsamically scented, frankincense contains sesquiterpenes, which enable it to go beyond the blood-brain barriers. In skin care, frankincense helps prevent scarring and aging and is used to smooth wrinkles.

Geranium: Not only is the rosy, lemony fragrance of geranium essential oil a pleasant scent in skin care combinations, it also has some impressive benefits. Geranium moisturizes dry skin, is suitable for sensitive skin, quiets wrinkles and makes skin supple. In addition, it helps in the healing of bruises, eczema, ringworm and shingles.

Helichrysum: Recognizable by its distinct, straw-like, honey aroma, helichrysum aids in the healing of bruises and psoriasis. It cleanses, reduces scarring and regenerates tissue.

Lavender: The qualities of this sweet, floral essential oil are beneficial in skin care. When added to carrier oil, it moisturizes dry skin, sensitive skin, skin ulcers, stretch marks and softens wrinkles. Lavender is comforting to sunburn and diabetic sores.

Lemongrass: As an effective skin care oil, lemongrass possesses healing properties that serve as an antiseptic and astringent for all skin types, resulting in healthy, glowing skin. It must be used with a carrier oil, as it can cause skin irritation. Lemongrass releases a grassy, pungent, lemony aroma.

Myrrh: Myrrh oil has a smoky, bitter odor. It holds terpenoids and sesquiterpenes both of which have anti-inflammatory and antioxidant effects. Sesquiterpenes help the user remain calm and balanced. In skin care, myrrh aids in healing chapped and cracked skin, skin ulcers, stretch marks, ringworm, weeping wounds and other skin conditions. In addition it smooths wrinkles. Among myrrh's qualities it is anti-infectious, anti-inflammatory, antiseptic, antitumor and astringent.

Sandalwood: Dry skin, acne, vitiligo, skin infection and skin regeneration can all benefit with the use of sandalwood essential oil. It gives off a woody, sweet fragrance.

Tea Tree: Also known as melaleuca, this oil emits a distinct, medicinal, herbaceous odor. Its cleansing properties benefit acne, cold sores, eczema, sunburn and warts.

Blend 1: Face All Aglow

2 drops Frankincense

3 drops Helichrysum

3 drops Lavender

2 drops Myrrh

2 drops Sandalwood

Jojoba

Add oils to a 10 ml dark-colored glass roller bottle or dropper bottle. Fill the remainder of the bottle with jojoba, leaving enough headspace for the roller ball or dropper. Shake lightly to mix oils. Smooth onto face to nourish the skin.

Blend 2: Naturally Young

3 drops Frankincense

4 drops Geranium

4 drops Lavender

3 drops Sandalwood

Add essential oils to your unscented facial lotion. Smooth gently onto your face. Avoid applying too close to eyes. This solution is used to reduce wrinkles and fine lines.

Blend 3: All Clear

4 drops Lavender

2 drops Lemongrass

4 drops Tea Tree

Jojoba

Drop the essential oils into a 10 ml dark-colored glass roller or dropper bottle. Fill the remainder of the bottle with jojoba, leaving enough headspace for the roller ball or dropper. You may need a small funnel to do this. When lid is secure, slightly shake the bottle to mix the oils. Apply to the face as needed. Store the bottle out of direct sunlight. If using a larger bottle, simply adjust the proportions as needed.

Blend 4: Better Butter

2 Tablespoons Beeswax

4 Tablespoons Jojoba

2 Tablespoons Shea Butter

6 Tablespoons Coconut Oil (not fractionated)

Lavender (optional)

Melt down beeswax and jojoba in a double boiler. When liquefied, stir in coconut oil until completely melted. Reduce heat and add shea butter, stirring mixture as it dissolves. Add coconut oil and stir until fully melted. Finally, add the shea butter, stirring as it melts. Pour the mixture into airtight glass jars or decorative airtight tins. If desired, gently stir in a drop or two of lavender essential oil. Replace the cover and allow mixture to cool. Apply liberally to affected areas as needed. This body butter can be used to protect and soften skin, soothe eczema and dry, itchy skin.

Summary

Department store shelves are chock-full of skin care products containing ingredients unhealthy to skin. By making your own skin care solutions, you will be the one deciding what will and will not be applied to your skin. Naturally, essential oils provide the health benefits your skin needs.

Chapter 3: Sweet Dreams

Being awakened by a baby's cry, and later waiting up for teenagers to come home after curfew has caused Alisa to be an insomniac. Even as an empty nester, she spent years wandering around the house, reading, writing, or finding something to do to make her drowsy. When introduced to a blend of essential oils for sleep, she had the first good night's sleep in a long time. If you ask her, she will tell you that the upside is that she awakens feeling rested and energetic. The downside is that her best creative writing happens in the wee hours of the night.

Everyone dreams of a good night's sleep. In this chapter we will discuss essential oils to help achieve this need.

Cedarwood: This warm, soft, woody, scented oil is calming and relieves tension

Lavender: Commonly used as a sleep aid, lavender relieves anxiety, stress, tension and promotes peaceful sleep. Its sweet, floral scent alone will find one drifting off.

Marjoram: Many people struggle with falling asleep, or staying asleep, because of restless leg syndrome, muscle tension, or leg cramps. Marjoram relieves these symptoms. It has a spicy, herbaceous essence.

Sandalwood: With its woody, sweet fragrance, sandalwood serves as an aphrodisiac and treats exhaustion and tension.

Ylang ylang: The sweet, tropical floral scent of ylang ylang is a favorite among many essential oil users. It is an aphrodisiacs, a sedative, is calming, relaxing and relieves exhaustion, stress and tension.

Blend 1: Alisa's "Go To" Blend

3 drops Lavender

2 drops Marjoram

2 drops Sandalwood

3 drops Ylang Ylang

1 scant Tablespoon Fractionated Coconut oil

Mix all together in a 10 ml dark-colored roller or dropper bottle. Fill the remainder of the bottle with fractionated coconut oil. Massage onto the bottoms of both feet before you slip into bed. Rub hands together to blend the oils into the palms. If you want to mix a larger amount all at once, use the same proportions. If the carrier oil is eliminated, you can halve the first four ingredients into a diffuser with water. This mixture creates a nice sleeping blend.

Blend 2: Calm Balm

5 drops Cedarwood

5 drops Lavender

Fractionated Coconut oil

Add oils to a 10 ml dark-colored glass roller or dropper bottle. Fill the remainder of the bottle with fractionated coconut oil, leaving enough headspace for the ball or dropper. Shake lightly to mix oils. To apply this concoction, roll on the bottoms of both feet and massage in.

Blend 3: Baby Blend

2 drops Lavender

1 teaspoon Fractionated Coconut oil

Children and infants relax when a few drops of lavender are mixed with a teaspoon of coconut oil and massaged into the bottoms of their feet.

If desired, combine water and lavender in a spritzer bottle and lightly mist over a child's pillow or teddy bear to help him sleep soundly as the sweet lavender smell lulls him off to sleep.

Blend 4: Rest in Peace

3 drops Lavender

4 drops Sandalwood

4 drops Ylang Ylang

Carrier oil of your choice

Add essential oils to a 10 ml dark-colored glass dropper bottle. Fill the remainder of the bottle with coconut oil. Shake slightly. This makes a soothing massage mixture for a relaxing sleep.

Summary

A plethora of essential oils aid in sleep. Give your favorites a try to find the combinations that work best for you. After a few weeks of using a blend of oils, they may temporarily lose their potency on you. Switch it up for a few weeks using a different solution. Alternating mixtures and methods may be helpful.

Chapter 4: Say No to Pain

For over a year, Bill looked up at the beautiful Bountiful temple that shone brightly on the mountain three miles up the hill from his apartment. Secretly, he set a goal that he would walk up that steep hill and back again, while he lived at the downtown apartment; the problem being that he had recently recovered from a knee injury. Actively working out at the gym, his strength, mobility and muscle mass were building. One evening, he set out with his wife intending to walk partially up the hill, hoping that eventually he could make it to the top. Before beginning the hike he slathered himself with a mixture of essential oils. As he walked, the oils worked into his joints, increasing his agility. Along the way he set mini-goals of how far they would walk. Higher, ever higher, they climbed. To his utter and complete excitement, that very evening, they found themselves standing on level ground with the beautiful temple on the hill.

Following are the essential oils mentioned in this chapter and the benefits they encompass.

Cardamom: Giving off both a sweet and spicy aroma, cardamom is used to relieve inflammation, muscle aches and sciatica.

Eucalyptus: This oil is used to soothe inflammation, sore muscles, over-exercised muscles and pain. Its fragrance is earthy, cooling and freshening.

Frankincense: Rich, warm and balsamically scented, frankincense contains sesquiterpenes, which enable it to go beyond the blood-brain barriers. It is used to relieve sciatic pain, soothe inflammation, promote healing, prevent scarring and to relieve a stress headache.

Ginger: Carrying a spicy, woody aroma, ginger is often used to relieve pain from arthritis, sore muscles, sprains and broken bones.

Juniper Berry: Juniper Berry smells piney, yet sweet. It soothes wounds, arthritis and aching muscles.

Lavender: This multi-tasking oil works where it is needed. Lavender relieves arthritis, inflammation, sprains and wounds. Its sweet, floral scent is calming, relaxing and sedative.

Peppermint: Minty, fresh and cooling, peppermint oil is used to calm charley horses, cramps, muscle aches and fatigue, sciatica, arthritis and inflammation.

Rosemary: Rosemary oil is often used to relax arthritis and inflammation pain. Its smell is sweet, fresh and penetrating.

Tea Tree: Also known as melaleuca, this oil emits a distinct, medicinal, herbaceous odor. Inflammation and wounds are often soothed with its use.

Wintergreen: The odor of wintergreen is strong, sweet and woody. It is used to quell pain in the bones, joints, rotator cuffs, as well as bring relief to frozen shoulder and arthritis.

Blend 1: Bill's Blend

4 drops Eucalyptus

4 drops Peppermint

2 drops Tea Tree

1 tablespoons Carrier oil of your choice

Blend oils together. Add 1 scant tablespoon of carrier oil. Carefully put mixture into a 10 ml dark-colored glass roller, or dropper bottle. Massage into your joints to relieve pain, taking care not to get oils into the eyes. If a larger bottle is used, simply adjust proportions as needed. Store the bottle away from direct sunlight. Be sure to use carrier oil, as these oils may be sensitive to the skin.

Blend 2: Oh, Pain!

Frankincense

Fractionated Coconut oil

Blend frankincense with coconut oil in a 50%/50% ratio. Add a little olive oil, if desired. Add to a dark-colored glass roller, or dropper bottle, leaving enough headspace for the roller ball or dropper. Store the bottle away from direct sunlight. Roll on desired location and massage into the skin. This mixture may also be used in the bath with a few drops of your favorite essential oils.

Blend 3: Back Attack

4 drops Cardamom

4 drops Ginger

4 drops Wintergreen

1 scant Tablespoon Extra Virgin Olive Oil

Blend all ingredients together to create a soothing massage oil. Use to relieve back pain, sore muscles and sciatica. Combine into a 10 ml dark-colored glass bottle.

Blend 4: Soothing Soak

2 drops Cypress

4 drops Juniper Berry

2 drops Lavender

2 drops Rosemary

1 squirt of Fractionated Coconut Oil

1 cup Epsom salts

After the tub is filled, add Epsom salt. Stir with your hand to help salts dissolve. Squirt the coconut oil into the tub and add the oils. Swirl water with your hand. Soak for a good 20 minutes or longer.

Summary

Back pain, joint pain, sciatica and arthritis are common complaints in a doctor's office. Patients want relief and they aren't very patient in waiting for it. Hopefully you will find some comfort in these methods and blends. Give them a try – what can it hurt?

Chapter 5: Don't Panic

During an abusive relationship, Julie felt flooded with feelings of stress. As a result, she suffered a mini-stroke which resulted in a blood clot, congestion on one side of her head and vision impairment. Although she wishes she had used essential oils to unruffled the built-up stress beforehand, she began using essential oils after finishing her medical treatments. Today the blood clot and congestion are gone, and some of her vision has returned.

Stress is an impulse we experience daily. We will learn ways to use essential oils to lessen our stress as we view recipes in this section. Each oil listed describes how it can help in coping with stress.

Bergamot: While both uplifting and refreshing, this sweet, citrusy oil relieves stress, aids with PMS symptoms and lifts the mood of its user. If using topically, avoid sunlight for 72 hours after applying.

Roman Chamomile: Chamomile is known for its calming, relaxing capabilities in adults and children alike. Its aroma is fresh, fruity and herbaceous.

Clary Sage: This oil emits a spicy, sharp, herbaceous odor. It has a soothing, sedative effect on the user of this oil.

Frankincense: Rich, warm and balsamically scented, frankincense contains sesquiterpenes, which enable it to go beyond the blood-brain barriers. It helps the user have a better attitude, relieves a stress headache and nervousness.

Lavender: Among the numerous benefits of this sweet, floral scented essential oil, it is calming, relieves stress, helps the user to control mood swings, crying, and to deal with sorrow more successfully.

Peppermint: Minty, fresh and cooling, this oil may be used to relieve stress headaches and to elevate mood.

Vetiver: Balsamic, with a heavy earthy smell, vetiver relieves stress and nervousness. It has also been used to help handle ADD/ADHD.

Ylang ylang: The sweet, tropical floral scent of ylang ylang is a favorite among many essential oil users. It is calming, relaxing, relieves exhaustion and stress. It may help the user deal with fearful situations.

Blend 1: Julie's Choice

5 drops Frankincense

5 drops Lavender

Carrier oil of your choice

Add oils to a 10 ml dark-colored glass roller bottle, or dropper bottle. Fill the remainder of the bottle with carrier oil, leaving enough headspace for the roller ball, or dropper. Shake lightly to mix oils. Apply to pulse points behind ears and on wrists. Rub wrists together and inhale the aroma.

Blend 2: Chill Out

2 drops Chamomile

2 drops Frankincense

2 drops Lavender

2 drops Peppermint

Carrier oil of your choice

For relaxation and stress headache relief, combine these mixed essential oils with a carrier oil and apply to your temples for a cooling effect.

Blend 3: Sleep Steep

1 teaspoon Bergamot

1 teaspoon Clary Sage

1 teaspoon Vetiver

1 squirt of Coconut oil

Add oils into a pre-filled tub. This mixture can be mixed with bath salts, Epsom salts, or bath oil. Soak at least 20 minutes to relax in preparation of a good night's sleep.

Blend 4: Clear the Air

2 drops Roman Chamomile

2 drops Lavender

2 drops Ylang Ylang

Diffuse in an essential oil friendly diffuser for calming and to relieve stress.

Summary

Don't be defeated by stress, rather experiment with essential oils, and methods, to find which treatment works best for you.

Chapter 6: Tummy Trouble

As long as Annie can remember, she has had stomach pain. For the most part, she has eliminated gluten, dairy and sugar from her diet, yet she still continues to bloat and complains of digestive issues. Recently, she began experimenting with essential oils. Annie has discovered a concoction that helps dismiss her stomach pain and controls the bloating. Below are some blends that may aid in digestion. Annie's favorite recipe follows the list of oils discussed.

Anise: If you know what black licorice smells like, you can well imagine the smell of anise. It is often used to reduce gas, bloating and to aid in digestion.

Caraway: Caraway can aid indigestion, settle an upset stomach and relieve colic, flatulence and gastric spasms. It gives off a pungent, anise-like aroma.

Cardamom: Giving off both a sweet and spicy aroma, cardamom is used to relieve nausea, flatulence and vomiting.

Chamomile: Roman Chamomile, known for its calming, relaxing capabilities in adults and children alike, will also help with colic, dysentery and stomach aches. Its aroma is fresh, fruity and herbaceous.

Coriander: Releasing a pleasing, fresh, spicy aroma, coriander is used to calm diarrhea, digestive spasms, flatulence and nausea.

Fennel: This earthy, sweet fragrant oil, similar to anise, is intended to improve digestion and to eliminate constipation, nausea, gastritis.

Frankincense: Rich, warm and balsamically scented, frankincense contains sesquiterpenes, which enable it to go beyond the blood-brain barriers. It helps with digestive distress, gastrointestinal discomfort and irritable bowel syndrome. It speeds up the digestion of food. Read the label of the bottle before ingesting. If it doesn't state that it can be taken internally please don't do it. Harmful effects may follow.

Ginger: Carrying a spicy, woody aroma, ginger aids in improving digestion, and suppresses diarrhea, flatulence, indigestion and nausea.

Peppermint: Minty, fresh and cooling, this oil is used to aid digestion, nullify constipation, diarrhea, gastritis, heartburn, indigestion, irritable bowel syndrome, nausea and vomiting.

Tarragon: This oil speeds up digestion by stimulating the secretion of digestive juices into the stomach, moving food through the whole digestive system. Tarragon emits a slightly spicy, green scent.

Blend 1: Annie's Answer

1 drop Fennel

1 drop Frankincense

1 drop Ginger

1 drop Peppermint

Carefully add oils into an empty gelatin capsule using a dropper. Take for indigestion when needed. These gel caps can be used three times a day. Several capsules can be made at a time, but store them in the refrigerator.

Blend 2: Belly Rub

2 drops Cardamom

2 drops Chamomile

2 drops Fennel

2 drops Ginger

2 drops Peppermint

1 scant Tablespoon Carrier oil of your choice

Drop oils into a dark-colored glass 10 ml roller, or dropper bottle. Using a small funnel, carefully pour carrier oil nearly to the top of the bottle, leaving a headspace for the roller ball, or dropper. When your stomach aches, roll oil over the back and abdomen, massaging in circular motions, being sure to smooth over the navel. You may also massage oils to the bottoms of your feet.

Blend 3: Gut Feeling

Anise

Caraway

Coriander

Fennel

Frankincense

Ginger

Peppermint

Tarragon

Add 4 or 5 drops of any combination of these oils to a diffuser filled with water to aid in digestive ailments.

Blend 4: Daily Digestion

1-3 drops Peppermint

This is an easy and inexpensive fix to aid in daily digestive health. Following are four ways you can accomplish this. 1) Add 1-3 drops of peppermint oil into a gelatin capsule and swallow it with a glass of water. 2) Mix 1-3 drops of peppermint into your daily drinking water or add to juice or a smoothie. 3) Diffuse 3 drops of peppermint in a diffuser filled with water. 4) Using the carrier oil of your choice, mix 1-3 drops of peppermint in the palm of your hand and rub it on your abdomen, back and/or bottoms of your feet. Pre-made gelatin capsules can be stored in the refrigerator.

Summary

Though nothing can replace good eating habits, exercise, and stress relief for good digestion, the recipes and methods of application may help calm digestive issues and help to improve the digestive tract.

Chapter 7: It's all in the Head

A crying, sick baby will keep a parent awake and active in the night, resulting in lack of sleep and usually an accompanying headache. James, committed to completing a piano refinishing project, was eager to try essential oils to help his tired, stress headache from intruding on his day. He was surprised to find that in a half an hour, or so, he was able to return to the task at hand. Of course, his baby slept most of the day, keeping the door wide open for another sleepless night for his parents. Though a variety of essential oils may help relieve a headache, we mention only a few in this chapter.

Roman Chamomile: Chamomile known for its calming, relaxing capabilities in adults and children alike will also help with insomnia. Its aroma is fresh, fruity and herbaceous.

Clove: The aroma of clove oil is spicy, bitter and woody. It calms fevers, tension headaches and sinusitis.

Eucalyptus: This oil is used to increase energy and to relieve fever and sinusitis. Its fragrance is earthy, cooling and freshening.

Frankincense: Rich, warm and balsamically scented, frankincense contains sesquiterpenes, which enable it to go beyond the blood-brain barriers. It helps a person have a better attitude, relieves a stress headache, tension and mental fatigue.

Lavender: This multi-tasking oil works where it is needed. Lavender calms headaches, migraines, nervous tension, stress, insomnia, exhaustion and pain. Its sweet, floral scent is calming, relaxing and sedative.

Myrrh: Myrrh oil has a smoky, bitter odor. It holds terpenoids and sesquiterpenes, both of which have anti-inflammatory and antioxidant effects. Sesquiterpenes help keep us calm and balanced. Among myrrh's qualities it is anti-infectious, anti-inflammatory, antiseptic, antitumor and astringent. Myrrh is often added to essential oil remedies for headaches.

Peppermint: Minty, fresh and cooling, this oil is used for chronic fatigue, fatigue, headaches, migraines, sinusitis and to elevate mood.

Rosemary: The fragrance of rosemary is sweet, fresh and penetrating. It carries analgesic, antibacterial, anticancer, anticatarrhal, antifungal, anti-infectious, anti-inflammatory, antioxidant and expectorant properties. Headaches and sinusitis may settle down while using.

Wintergreen: The odor of wintergreen is strong, sweet and woody. It is used to reduce pain and fevers.

Blend 1: James' Choice

2 drops Frankincense

2 drops Lavender

2 drops Peppermint

2 drops Rosemary

2 drops Wintergreen

1 scant Tablespoon Sweet Almond oil

Drop oils into a dark-colored glass 10 ml roller or dropper bottle. Using a small funnel, carefully pour sweet almond oil nearly to the top of the bottle, leaving a headspace for the roller ball or dropper. When headache attacks, roll oil over the temples, forehead, back of neck and to the bottoms of feet. Store oil in a cool, dark place.

Blend 2: Sit 'n' Soak

2 drops Chamomile

1 drop Clove

3 drops Lavender

4 drops Wintergreen

1 cup Epsom Salt

1 squirt Fractionated Coconut oil

After tub is filled, dump in the Epsom salt and drip the oils into the tub. Swoosh the water with your hand to distribute oil. Add a squirt of coconut oil. Enjoy this therapeutic bath for at least 20 minutes.

Blend 3: Head to Head

 2 drops Eucalyptus

1 drop Myrrh

3 drops Peppermint

This mixture can either be added with water to a diffuser, or used as either a cold or warm compress. For a cold compress, add the oils to one quart cool or icy water. Soak a clean cloth in the bowl. Wring out excess water and apply to forehead or back of neck. Use the same process for a warm compress using a comfortable temperature of heat. A cold compress usually works best, but to improve circulation, it may help to alternate between cold and warm.

Blend 4: Head Rush

2 drops Chamomile

2 drops Lavender

1 teaspoon Fractionated Coconut oil

As soon as you recognize that a headache is on its way, cup your palm and mix all ingredients together with your finger. Massage the oil to your temples, forehead and back of neck. If possible, rub onto the bottom of your feet, as well.

Summary

Headaches accompany illnesses, allergies and also come from stress or sleepless nights. If you can determine the type of headache, you can use these methods of relief and review the book to look for treatments of the ailment you may be suffering.

Chapter 8: A Breath of Fresh Air

In the past, Clint's drain tubes became clogged whenever he got sick. Lumps formed on the sides of his neck, just below the ear, where infection collected. These lumps had been known to be the size of a baseball. This condition occurred about twice a year, lasting 6–8 weeks at a time. Occasionally, he ended up at the hospital where a doctor had to cut into him to drain the infection. By the time he was introduced to essential oils, he was desperate. Today, when he feels the lumps starting to form, he uses a mucus rub. He hasn't had a lump for three years. Below the list of essential oils that may help with respiratory ailments, you will find the recipe that Clint uses.

Cypress: Asthma, fever, nose bleeds, flu, pain, swollen eyes and throat problems can be addressed with the fresh, evergreen aroma of cypress.

Eucalyptus: Asthma, bronchitis, ear inflammation, congestion, cough, fever, flu, hay fever, respiratory viruses and sinusitis have been relieved with eucalyptus. Its fragrance is earthy, cooling and freshening.

Lavender: This multi-tasking oil works where it is needed. Lavender calms allergies, asthma, bronchitis, earaches, fever, flu, hay fever, headaches, pain and respiratory problems. Its sweet, floral scent is calming, relaxing and sedative.

Lemon: Used often in flavoring, this clean, uplifting, citrusy oil relieves colds, fever, flu, respiratory problems, sore throat, tonsillitis and pain.

Marjoram: Acting as an expectorant, marjoram eases colds and headaches. It has a spicy, herbaceous essence.

Myrtle: Clear, herbaceous and freshly scented, myrtle is an expectorant and supports the respiratory system. It is also sedative in nature.

Peppermint: Minty, fresh and cooling, this oil is used to treat congestion, flu, headaches, sinusitis and throat infection.

Ponderosa pine: What does it smell like? Why, camping, of course, or a hike through the forest. It serves as a pain reliever and is known for its respiratory capabilities.

Rosemary: The fragrance of rosemary is sweet, fresh and penetrating. It carries analgesic, antibacterial, anticancer, anticatarrhal, antifungal, anti-infectious, anti- inflammatory, antioxidant and expectorant properties. Flu, headaches and sinusitis are quieted with Rosemary.

Spruce: Spruce expels a fresh, clean, forest fragrance. Promotes clear, smooth breathing and fights congestion.

Tea Tree: Also known as melaleuca, this oil emits a distinct, medicinal, herbaceous odor. Its cleansing properties benefit allergies, bronchitis, colds, coughs, itchy eyes, ear infections, earaches, sore throats, staph infections, bacterial and viral infections.

Blend 1: Clint's Concoction

2 drops Cypress

4 drops Eucalyptus Radiata

2 drops Lavender

2 drops Marjoram

3 drops Myrtle

2 drops Peppermint

4 drops Ponderosa Pine

2 drops Spruce

2 drops Tea Tree

Fractionated Coconut oil

Mix all oils together in a one ounce, dark-colored glass roller, or dropper bottle. Massage onto the chest, behind ears, and on the pads of toes and feet. Roll onto wrists and rub them together. Inhale.

Blend 2: Four Seasons

3 drops Lavender

3 drops Lemon

3 drops Peppermint

Carrier oil

Combine oils in a dark-colored glass 10 ml roller or dropper bottle. Store bottle out of direct sunlight. Roll onto the pulse points behind ears and wrists, then rub wrists together and inhale. This can also be massaged onto the chest and the pads of toes and feet.

Blend 3: Seasonal Trio

2 drops Lavender

2 drops Lemon

2 drops Peppermint

Drop all 6 drops together into a gel capsule. Take up to three times daily. These capsules can be pre-made and stored in the refrigerator.

Blend 4: Bath Bombs/Shower Melts

Ice cube tray, mini works best

2 cup Cornstarch

6 drops Eucalyptus Oil

2 drops Lemon

2 drops Peppermint

2 drops Rosemary

Food Coloring (optional)

4 Tablespoons water

Measure the cornstarch into a bowl. Add the essential oils. Mix well. The mixture will be crumbly. Add a few drops of food coloring, if desired, and continue to mix well. Slowly add in the four Tablespoons of water. Continue to mix until colors blend in and clumps begin to form. Add more water, a little at a time, until you have a thick paste. Scoop the mixture into a mini ice cube tray. Smooth each section out flat. Freeze for one hour or until set. Toss a bath bomb into the tub for a therapeutic bath. For the shower, place the bomb on a shallow soap dish. The hot water and shower steam will melt the bomb and diffuse the therapeutic aroma. If the unused bombs hold their shape they can be stored in a cool, dry place. If they are too runny, they can be stored in the freezer.

Summary

Whether you suffer with summer allergies to grass, hay, plants and pollen, or colds and flu in the winter months, these recipes will hopefully alleviate your respiratory problems.

Chapter 9: A Fungus Among Us

In the introduction of this book, I revealed the incident that led me to welcome the power of essential oils: the smashed thumb that remained marred for years, allowing a nasty fungus to grow inside of my nail. Following the list of essential oils mentioned in this chapter, I will unveil the concoction that aided in the healing of my thumb.

Frankincense: Rich, warm and balsamically scented, frankincense contains sesquiterpenes, which enable it to go beyond the blood-brain barriers. Its healing abilities are used to treat the herpes simplex virus, infected wounds and staph infection.

Lavender: This multi-tasking oil works where it is needed. Lavender relieves itching and pain, and can aid in the healing of cold sores, wounds and other skin conditions. Its sweet, floral scent is calming, relaxing and sedative.

Marjoram: Though fungus and viral infections are hard to treat, marjoram aids in the healing of these infections. It is used for cold sores, ringworm, sores and pain. It has a spicy, herbaceous essence.

Melissa: Melissa has a unique, pleasant, delicate, citrusy fragrance. Among its valuable uses, it aids in the healing of cold sores and viral infections.

Rosemary: The fragrance of rosemary is sweet, fresh and penetrating. It carries analgesic, antibacterial, anticancer, anticatarrhal, antifungal, anti-infectious, anti- inflammatory, antioxidant and expectorant properties.

Tea Tree: Also known as melaleuca, this oil emits a distinct, medicinal, herbaceous odor. Its cleansing properties benefit cold sores, pink eye, itchy eyes, ringworm, fungal infections, viral infections, candida and warts.

My Tried and True Anti-Fungal Blend:

3 drops Frankincense

3 drops Lavender

2 drops Sweet Marjoram

2 drops Rosemary

3 drops Tea Tree oil

1/2 teaspoon Extra Virgin Olive oil

1/2 Tablespoon Jojoba

To a 10 ml dark-colored glass roller, or dropper bottle, add the essential oils. Next add extra virgin olive oil. Lastly, fill the remainder of the bottle with jojoba leaving a small headspace to insert the roller ball, or dropper. A small funnel will make this process easier. When the lid is secure, slightly shake mixture to combine oils. Apply 3 or 4 times a day. Between applications, treat problem area with a drop of tea tree directly onto fungus. An additional drop of frankincense added directly on fungus once a day is also preferred. Continue treatment for a month, or longer, after the fungus has cleared to be sure it has been wiped out. A small funnel will make the transfer easier. When the lid is secure, slightly shake the mixture to combine oils. Apply 4 or 5 times a day. Keep using for a month after fungus is gone to make sure it has been healed.

Cold Sore (fever blister) Blend:

1 drop Lavender

1 drop Marjoram

1 drop Melissa

1 drop Tea Tree

1 teaspoon Apple Cider Vinegar

Combine oils and store in a small, dark-colored bottle that is easily accessible for outbreaks. This blend makes a powerful astringent. At the first tingling sensation preceding a developing cold sore, immediately begin using this solution. Apply directly to cold sore frequently until healed. Do not apply to broken skin.

Pink Eye (conjunctivitis) Blend:

2 drops Lavender

2 drops Tea Tree

1 teaspoon Extra Virgin Olive Oil

Before treating, blot eye with a warm, damp wash cloth to clean out any congestion or gunk. Throw the cloth in the hamper. Do not reuse wash cloth before laundering. Mix oils together in the palm of your hand. Massage along the base of your neck, and along both cheek bones, taking care not to get into the eyes. At bedtime, massage into the pads of both feet. Whether the conjunctivitis is of the viral, bacterial or allergy form, this should alleviate it.

Ringworm Blend:

2 drops Lavender

1 drop Marjoram

2 drops Tea Tree

1 teaspoon Extra Virgin Olive Oil

After mixing oils together into the palm of your hand, apply to affected area with a cotton swab. Do not reuse the swab. This solution may also be applied to the bottoms of your feet to help prevent the condition from spreading to other areas of the body.

Summary

Cold sores, fungi, pink eye and ringworm are highly contagious conditions. For best treatment, catch them early before they spread to neighboring body parts. The blends above may help to lessen their duration.

Chapter 10: Pests - The Uninvited Guests

Mike and Ruth enjoy their summer cabin near the lake. Their family congregates for swimming, boating, fishing and roasting marshmallows by the campfire. Unfortunately, the rodents liked to congregate, too. Rats attempted to enter the cabin by eating the wooden threshold. Ruth discovered holes where mice were coming into the cabin. With essential oils, they were able to keep the rats from the threshold and the mice outside.

Following are essential oils that will be discussed in this section.

Catnip: Catnip is often used to repel mosquitoes, house flies, mites, cockroaches, ticks and aphids. Be careful where you put it though, it will attract cats, and even put your house cat in a tizzy.

Cedarwood: Though this warm, soft, woody, scented oil is beneficial to humans, it is lethal to mosquitos, ticks and fleas.

Cinnamon: The warm, sweet, spirited fragrance and flavor of this oil will repel mosquitos. When applying to skin, never use more than 1% cinnamon oil to 99% liquid. For patio or home use, the maximum dilution is ¼ teaspoon per 4 ounces of liquid.

Citronella: Derived from lemongrass, citronella is very efficient at repelling insects. It also serves as an antiseptic to clean and treat insect bites.

Citrus oils: Any of the citrus oils, or a combination, may be used to deter ants. These oils are phototoxic, however, and may cause sun sensitivity to human skin.

Clove: The aroma of clove oil is spicy, bitter and woody. It repels insects and termites. To relieve bites and stings be sure to mix with a carrier oil.

Lemon Eucalyptus: While its fragrance is earthy, cooling and refreshing, the smell disorients mosquitos, thus repelling them. It doubles as an antiseptic after insect bites. It is also used to treat lice.

Lavender: Surprisingly enough, this sweet floral scent repels gnats, midges, mosquitos, ticks and fleas. It is also the "go to" oil to soothe bites and stings.

Lemongrass: Lemongrass is known for its ability to repel insects and fleas. It has a grassy, pungent, lemony aroma. It can cause skin irritation, so be sure to use with a carrier oil when applying to skin.

Neem: Neem oil is growing in popularity in its natural ability to repel insects, mosquitos, fleas, ticks and spiders.

Marjoram: Though fungus and viral infections are hard to treat, marjoram aids in the healing of these infections. It is used for cold sores, ringworm, sores and pain. It has a spicy, herbaceous essence.

Rosemary: Its sweet, fresh, penetrating smell repels mosquitos, flies and fleas. It is also used to treat lice.

Spearmint: The pleasant minty, fruity smell of spearmint oils serves as an insecticide. It fends off mosquitos, gnats, moths, flies and other flying insects.

Tea Tree: Insects, ticks, spiders and mites detest the medicinal, herbaceous odor of this oil.

Blend 1: Ruth's Revenge

(Mice/Insect Deterrent)

Peppermint or Clove oil

Mothballs or Cotton balls

Douse a mothball or cotton ball with peppermint, or clove, and place strategically around the house where the pests come in.

Mice and insects abhor the smell of peppermint. In a few weeks, as the odor dissipates, refresh the cotton balls.

Blend 2: Ants – Go Marching

Cinnamon (Not more than ¼ teaspoon per 4 oz. water)

Citrus oils (your choice)

Clove

Eucalyptus

Peppermint

Add about 20 drops of essential oils with water into a small squirt bottle. Either use single oil or a mixture of oils. Spray ant trails and entrance points. Reapplication may be needed after it dries.

Blend 3: Spider Chase

10 drops of Citrus, Lavender, Neem, Peppermint or Tea Tree

Liquid dish soap

Warm water

Directions

Put 10 drops of essential oil in a spray bottle. You can use individual oil or a combination of oils. Fill with water leaving a head space for the spray nozzle. Add a squirt of dish soap. After screwing on the nozzle, shake the mixture. Using the hose attachment, vacuum spider webs, egg sacs, and along carpet edges. Finally, spray mixture around window frames, along doorways, heat vents and all other places a spider might find comfortable.

Blend 4: Home Security

3 oz. Vinegar

3 oz. Water

15 drops of Essential oils

Fill an 8 ounce glass spray bottle with half vinegar and half water, leaving a headspace for the spray nozzle. Experiment with these oils and a variety of mixtures: citronella, clove, eucalyptus, lavender, lemongrass, peppermint, spearmint and tea tree.

Recipe 5: Bug Off

3 oz. Distilled or boiled Water

3 oz. Soybean Oil or Witch Hazel

10 drops Citronella

10 drops Clove

10 drops Eucalyptus

10 drops Lemongrass

10 drops Peppermint

Fill an 8 ounce spray bottle with distilled, or boiled, water and soybean oil, or witch hazel, nearly to the top, leaving a headspace for the sprayer. Drop in the essential oils. For a stronger spray, add more oils. Spray onto body and clothing. Other oils you can experiment with are cedarwood, catnip, tea tree oil, lavender, rosemary and cinnamon, in a variety of combinations. If using cinnamon, never use more than 1% cinnamon oil to 99% liquids.

Summary

There are many harmful chemicals on the market today to rid us of our unwanted guests. Hopefully, you will find a combination of essential oils that will safely replace these household hazards.

Conclusion

In the researching, experimenting and writing of this book, I am reminded how much I delight in essential oils. I use them daily and am always on the ready when a guest comes to my house with an ailment. These precious oils are my medicinal arsenal. The world around us is beautiful in all of its glory and splendor. Whether you are a naturalist, a spiritualist, or someone who dislikes adding chemicals to your body, I hope you learn to love essential oils, and their benefits, as much as I do.

This past Thanksgiving, as my family arrived for our celebration, the tangy fragrance of diffusing citrus oils welcomed them inside my home. At dinner, many family members complimented the tasty kick of the stuffing. I didn't tell them that I seasoned the bread cubes with a few drops of basil, marjoram, oregano and thyme oils. Nor did I tell them that I added clove and cinnamon oils to the perfectly spiced, homemade pumpkin pie. The zesty addition of orange oil to the traditional cranberry sauce was especially pleasing to the palate. Conflict, contention and hurt feelings often accompany our family gatherings. Not this time. We enjoyed being around each other. A calm, peaceable feeling enveloped the room. Everyone got along well: even the children.

Carrier Oils Used in this Book

Sweet Almond Oil: Brimming with vitamins A, B and E, almond oil increases circulation, protects against UV rays, and smooths wrinkles and fine lines. It is healthy for hair and nails. Massage therapists find that it glides easily over skin and is silky enough to add moisture and nourishment without being too oily. People with nut allergies should not use sweet almond oil. Buy only in small quantities, since it has a short shelf life.

Apple Cider Vinegar: As an old housewife's remedy, the acidity in vinegar may dry out a cold sore; prevent acne and works well in natural bug spray. Containing anti-bacterial, anti-inflammatory and anti-oxidant properties, it is an astringent, a disinfectant and balances the body's pH levels. Vitamins, minerals, enzymes, carbolic acid, ketones, aldehydes, amino acids, dietary fiber and acetic acid are all part of its composition.

Beeswax: In aromatherapy, beeswax is popular in the making of cosmetics, lip balms, butters, lotions and candles. Mainly it is used to help the products thicken and solidify. Containing anti-bacterial and antiseptic properties and vitamin A, it is an excellent emollient, skin softener and skin soother. Its fragrance is of honey and flower pollen.

Fractionated Coconut Oil: You will not find this version of coconut oil in your kitchen cupboard. Fractionated coconut oil will stay light, liquid and non-greasy all year long. It spreads well for topical application with no noticeable aroma. Fractionated coconut oil absorbs well, leaving skin feeling moisturized. This oil doesn't stain sheets as some carriers have been known to do. It also has a long shelf life.

Coconut Oil (not fractionated): Though the health benefits of coconut oil are the same as the fractionated version, this form is used in cosmetics and lotions so that the oil will harden up at room temperature.

Epsom Salt: In water, Epsom salt breaks down into magnesium and sulfate. Dissolving it in warm bath water can help relax muscles and loosen stiff joints. It is used for arthritis pain and swelling, bruises and sprains, fibromyalgia, ingrown toenails, insomnia, psoriasis, sunburn, and itchy red, swollen feet. It is often used in physical therapy for injured muscles, joints and other ailments.

Jojoba: Jojoba is actually a wax ester packed with vitamins B and E and contains antibacterial and anti-inflammatory properties. Though it has a gentle smell, it takes on the essence of the oils that are added to it. The use of it alone encourages healthy vibrant skin, but the result is compounded when mixed with essential oils. It is used for dandruff, dry skin, acne, wrinkles, to brighten dark spots on the skin and to minimize the appearance of pores. Jojoba, ideal for all skin conditions, is a quality carrier with an indefinite shelf life.

Extra Virgin Olive Oil: Popular and easy to find, extra virgin olive oil has a stronger aroma than most carrier oils. It is also thicker and leaves an oily feeling on the skin. Often it is combined with another carrier oil to dilute it, yet add its benefits. Full of proteins, vitamins and minerals, olive oil is calming for rheumatic conditions. It has as short shelf life of 18 months.

Sesame Seed Oil: Though this oil is thick in consistency and leaves an oily film on the skin, it is often combined with another carrier oil to dilute it, and to add its properties. Sesame oil is good for anxiety, bloating, constipation, excessive dryness, poor circulation, psoriasis and eczema. It contains antioxidants, vitamin E, protein, lecithin and minerals. Among its qualities, it is anti-bacterial, anti-fungal, anti-viral and anti-inflammatory. Shelf life: 1 year.

Shea Butter: Though it is not a carrier oil, its natural properties make it suitable for aromatherapy purposes. Shea butter is mainly used in the making of cosmetics and for some medicinal ointments. Its smooth, creamy texture is highly moisturizing making it popular in massage blends, lotions and other skin care products. It emits a nutty, fatty aroma and has a shelf-life of two years. People with nut allergies should ask a physician before using shea butter.

Soybean oil: Soybean oil, high in vitamins A, B, E, and lecithin is a favorable massage oil, suitable for all types of skin, producing a smooth texture and luxurious feel. It stays supple and is very light on the skin and carries a very light scent. Benefits include improvement of the quality of skin, hair and glands. It is popularly used in making cosmetics, lotions, soap and anti-aging solutions. Shelf life: 6 months to a year. Refrigerate after opening.

Sunflower Oil: Rich in vitamin E, fatty acid, linoleic acid, palitic acid and stearic acid, this oil benefits the skin. It is light, non-greasy and penetrates well without leaving an oily residue. It has a faint, sweet aroma. Most commonly it is used in massage oils, body lotions and body oils. To keep from going rancid, store sunflower oil in a cool, dark place. Shelf life: 12 months.